Aromatherapy for Beginners: Getting Started with Essential Oils

Written by Aimee Anderson

This book contains material protected under International and Federal Copyright Laws and Treaties. Any unauthorized reprint or use of this material is prohibited. No part of this book may be reproduced or transmitted in any form or by any means, electronic or mechanical, including photocopying, recording, or by any information storage and retrieval system without express written permission from the author.

I0428634

Disclaimer:

The information contained in this book is for general information purposes only.

While we endeavor to keep the information up to date and correct, we make no representations or warranties of any kind, express or implied, about the completeness, accuracy, reliability, suitability or availability with respect to the book or the information, products, services, or related graphics contained in the book for any purpose. Any reliance you place on such information is therefore strictly at your own risk.

None of the information in this this book is meant to be construed as medical advice. Always consult with a medical professional prior to making any changes in your life.

None of the health benefits mentioned in this book pertaining to use of essential oils have been evaluated or approved by the FDA. Do not use essential oils in place of medical treatment, nor should they be used to treat, diagnose, cure or prevent any disease, ailment or injury. Use essential oils at your own risk.

Contents

Introduction

Thank you for purchasing this book. It's designed with beginners to the world of essential oils in mind, but there's a lot of good information inside and it's a good refresher course no matter what your experience level is.

Some of the topics covered in this book include what essential oils are and why they're important, the best ways to use essential oils and essential oil safety. We also cover applications for a number of the more popular essential oils on the market today.

Thanks again for purchasing this book. I hope you enjoy reading it as much I enjoyed writing it!

Essential Oils and Aromatherapy

Essential oils are oils that are contained within all parts of a plant. While essential oil is the most common term used to refer to plant oils, they're also called ethereal oils, volatile oils or they're referred to as the oil of the specific plant they came from. These oils can be taken from all types of plants, including flowers, trees, shrubs and bushes.

The flowers, leaves and stems usually contain larger amounts of oil, but it can be found within the heartwood, branches, bark, roots and seeds of the plant. Oils can also be extracted from the resins, gums and saps of plants using a number of innovative distillation techniques. The chemical composition of the oil can vary depending on what part of the plant it was extracted from, where the plant was grown, the conditions under which it was grown and a number of other factors.

There are several methods used to extract essential oils from plants. They can be distilled using steam, water or centrifugal force, or the plants can be crushed and the oil can be collected. Some oils are extracted through use of solvents, but these oils are generally avoided for aromatherapy purposes because some of the solvent may be left behind.

While there are a growing number of people who consider these oils essential to their daily lives, essential oils get the "essential" portion of their name from the fact that they're essential to the plants they come from. They play a number of roles within these plants, ranging from keeping predators at bay to preventing other plants from taking root and growing in the soil nearby.

Here are just some of the many actions essential oils are responsible for while contained within the plants they're derived from:

- **Keeping pests from attacking the plant.**
- **Attracting pollinating insects to the plant.**
- **Attracting predatory insects that will prey on pests.**
- **Keeping plants in good health.**
- **Fighting disease.**
- **Preventing fungal or bacterial growth.**
- **Preventing other plants and weeds from taking root in the soil around the plant.**

The aromatic essences of plants don't just benefit the plants they come from, they carry with them some definite benefits for humans as well. Man has known for tens of thousands of years that certain plants carry great power when it comes to health and wellness. From ancient times to modern day, a number of plants and their oils have been employed to treat all sorts of illnesses and ailments. While our ancestors undoubtedly viewed these plants with reverence and awe, often believing they carried magical powers, we now know there are a vast number of compounds inside the plants that are beneficial to the human body.

These compounds include aldehydes, alcohols, phenols, esters, ethers, terpenes and ketones, just to name a few. The more complex the blend of aromatic compounds, the more intense and exotic the oil smells and the more beneficial the oil becomes. These compounds meld together to give a plant its characteristic fragrance and in doing so creates an oil that can carry with it a number of therapeutic properties.

For many years, plants and their oils were the only sensible option for treating all sorts of physical and mental ailments, but in modern times they've fallen out of favor in lieu of Western medicine. Now, instead of turning to natural compounds to help heal our bodies, we instead turn to chemicals that are often designed to mask problems instead of helping prevent them. Some of these chemicals work well and modern medicine has definite benefits, but it doesn't always have to be the answer, especially for minor issues that don't threaten life and limb.

A large number of people are turning to essential oils and aromatherapy treatments to enhance their physical, mental and even spiritual well-being. These oils can be used on their own or they can be combined to create powerful oil blends that contain a number of beneficial compounds. The right blend of oils, when inhaled or applied to the skin, has the power to release chemicals within the brain that can alter your mood, and essential oils have the ability to enter the blood stream and to travel throughout the body, taking action everywhere they go.

We'll cover the many beneficial actions these oils take in future chapters, but for now just be aware no matter how they're applied, be it through diffusion, inhalation or topical application, they can travel through the blood stream to other areas of the body, including the internal organs and the brain.

The Benefits of Aromatherapy

Aromatherapy is one of those things you can go a lifetime without using, but once you learn about essential oils and how to use them to your benefit, you'll wonder how you ever lived without them. Essential oils have a number of uses, ranging from improving one's health and emotional well-being to household cleaning and sanitization. As long as you take care to avoid oils that are distilled using solvents or that have been *adulterated*, meaning they've been diluted with other compounds, essential oils are entirely natural. Instead of bombarding your body with unnatural compounds it doesn't recognize, you're using natural compounds your body was designed by nature to take in and process.

Don't take this to mean essential oils aren't powerful compounds and can be used in any manner you'd like. They're extremely powerful and caution should be taken when applying essential oils or you could end up doing more harm than good. That said, when essential oils are safely and properly applied, they carry with them a number of benefits and can be used as an organic and holistic approach to treatment of a variety of conditions. While they'll likely never be able to replace modern medicine, they can be used in conjunction with modern medicine to help ease a number of conditions and ailments. Always consult with your physician before attempting to use essential oils to treat any health condition you may be suffering. Essential oils are powerful and there may be contraindications you aren't aware of.

Essential oils contain a number of natural chemical compounds that are beneficial to the human body. Here's a small sampling of the many benefits of essential oils:

- **They kill bacteria and fungus and prevent them from growing.**
- **They prevent sepsis in wounds.**
- **They reduce external and internal inflammation.**
- **They eliminate oxidants.**
- **They soothe aches and pains.**
- **Viral infections can be eliminated.**
- **The immune system gets a boost.**
- **They cause the brain to release "feel good" chemicals.**
- **They can be used to boost energy and to keep the user alert.**
- **They can be used to lessen symptoms associated with the flu and the common cold.**
- **Respiratory conditions including congestion and coughing can be eased with certain oils.**
- **Circulation is improved.**
- **Skin health can be improved.**
- **Certain oils can be used to improve dental health.**

Keep in mind this is just a partial list, designed to give you an idea of how powerful essential oils really are. No single oil features all of these benefits, but you can create powerful oil blends that allow you to combine the many benefits of a number of oils.

While essential oils have definite benefits when it comes to improving one's health, perhaps of greater benefit is their ability to alter the mind. They can be used to change bad moods into good, sadness into happiness and stress into relaxation. Some people are even able to use them in conjunction with professional therapy to help them find relief from depression and feelings of distress.

Be aware that scientists are just now starting to unlock the secrets of essential oils and a number of the claims made about the uses of essential oils are based on anecdotal evidence. While there's likely some truth to many of these claims, those facing severe health issues and major medical emergencies should never attempt to use aromatherapy as treatment for their ailments. Use common sense and practice aromatherapy when it's appropriate.

Purchasing Essential Oils

There are hundreds of places you can purchase essential oils from, both in person and online. They're found in health food stores, beauty supply shops and lately they've even been popping up in grocery stores and large retailers. Perhaps the best place to source essential oils is online, but you're going to want to do a little bit of research before making a purchase. Look for trusted companies that are recommended by other people. Some brands are good, some are bad and some are big unknowns. Essential oils aren't heavily regulated by the government and there's little to no oversight in regards to what's actually in bottles labeled as essential oil, so it's important to properly vet any company you're thinking about using before making a purchase.

Many companies grade their oils, labeling them with titles like "therapeutic grade," "medicinal grade," or any of a number of other terms. Be aware these labels are meaningless in the grand scheme of things because they're made up by the manufacturer in an attempt to make their essential oil brand stand out from the crowd.

The best essential oils for aromatherapy purposes are pure, unadulterated organic oils, but determining whether an oil meets those standards may not be as simple as looking at the label. There are companies out there that take expensive oils and adulterate them, adding less expensive oils, which is bad, or synthetic fragrances, which is even worse, to the more-expensive oils to dilute them so they can make more money. This is a common practice with high-end oils like rose otto oil and isn't a problem when the oils are properly labeled. When a bottle is labeled as an *oil blend,* it usually means other essential oils have been used to dilute the more expensive oil. Oils labeled as *absolute* have been diluted with something else. Oil blends are usually fine to use for aromatherapy, but absolutes are to be avoided unless you feel you absolutely have to have the expensive oil and can't afford the unadulterated version. Excuse the pun.

It's always exciting to find a great deal on essential oils, but beware of deals that seem too good to be true. If you know the average price of an oil is high and you find it on sale for a rock-bottom price, it's time to step back and question whether the deal is indeed too good. Oils that are difficult to obtain are always going to command a high price and there isn't much manufacturers can do to lower the price of pure oil. Cut-rate sellers may be adulterating the oil and selling it as pure or they may be selling something completely different than what's on the label.

The Difference between Essential Oils and Perfumes

Since they both smell good, it's all too easy to get essential oils and perfumes mixed up. People tend to want to group them in the same group even though chemically they're very different from one another. Further compounding the matter is the fact that some high-end perfumes do contain small amounts of expensive essential oils to enhance their fragrance.

The key difference between essential oils and perfumes is that most perfumes are made using synthetic fragrances. These fragrances smell good and can often be tailor-made to mimic the scents of essential oils, but the similarities stop there. Synthetic fragrances are produced to keep costs down and the bottom line high, but they don't feature the same beneficial compounds that are found in essential oils. Their benefits stop at the good smell.

Even when essential oils are used in perfumes, they don't carry the same benefits as they normally would because they've more often than not been diluted with chemical compounds. Never attempt to use perfume in lieu of essential oils unless all you want to do is smell good.

Essential Oil Applications

Aromatherapy practitioners deliver essential oils to the body in two basic ways. The oils are applied directly to the skin or the fragrance of the oils is inhaled.

When essential oils are applied topically, they're absorbed directly into the skin and can be used to help take care of skin conditions, aches and pains, cramping and a number of other localized issues. They soak into the skin, where they're picked up by the small capillaries resting just below the surface and are transported throughout the body. Essential oils applied topically don't just affect the area where they're applied. Once they make it into the bloodstream, they benefit the entire body. You can rub the oil blend into a specific area of your body or you can have a partner massage it into a larger area.

Most essential oils need to be diluted with carrier oil prior to application. Add a few drops of essential oil or your favorite blend of essential oils to a tablespoon of carrier oil and blend it in before applying it to the skin. There are only a handful of oils that can be applied *neat*, which is the term used to denote undiluted application of essential oil.

Another method used to topically apply essential oils is to add several drops to the bathtub. It's best to add them directly into the water stream while the tub is filling in order to disperse them throughout the water column. The essential oil will eventually float to the top of the water and will coat your body as you get out of the tub. This technique is best used with mild oils like lavender oil. Make sure you test any oil you plan on adding to the tub by applying a tiny amount to an inconspicuous area of your body prior to getting into a bathtub with essential oil added.

Diffused or inhaled essential oils take similar action on the body to oils that are applied topically, with a couple key differences. When you breathe the fragrance of essential oils in, tiny particles of oil are inhaled and will land on the soft tissues in your nose and respiratory system. These tiny particles are absorbed into the body and make their way into the bloodstream. Additionally, when you breathe in the aroma of the essential oils, the brain registers the fragrance of the oil and begins to release beneficial chemicals into the body as a result. This impacts your emotional state of mind and can leave you feeling calm and relaxed or stimulated and ready to take on the world, depending on which oils are used.

In order to administer essential oils via inhalation, the oils need to be diffused into the air. The following methods can all be used to get the fragrance of essential oil into the air:

- **Electric diffusers.** There are a number of commercial diffusers that are designed to break the oil into tiny particles and disperse it into the room. Electric diffusers are effective, but be careful not to use one that heats the oil because it can damage sensitive compounds in the oils.
- **Atomizers and nebulizers.** These machines are highly-effective because they break essential oils up into tiny particles that quickly fill all but the largest of the rooms. Thick oils can clog up these machines.

- **Clay pots and reed diffusers.** These simple diffusion tools use porous clay pots or pots with wooden rods in them to diffuse essential oil.

Of course, you can always keep it simple and add a few drops of essential oil to a napkin and hold it up to your nose or you can just open the bottle and breathe the fragrance of the oil in. When using essential oils to help with respiratory conditions, fill your sink with hot water, add several drops of essential oil to the water and hold your face over the sink while breathing deeply.

Other applications of essential oils include adding them to natural dental care, skin care and even hair care products to improve their effectiveness. Blending essential oils into these products allows you to up the therapeutic benefits of the product while making them smell great. Speaking of smelling great, essential oils can also be added to a spray bottle full of water and sprayed into rooms with odors you want to get rid of. This same spray can be used in the fridge to clean and deodorize it. It can also be used to deodorize stinky shoes, backpacks and many other items that smell bad. The best part is it doesn't just cover the smell; it completely eliminates it. A few drops added to the rinse cycle of your dishes will leave them sparkling and smelling great and you can even add them to your fabric softener to leave your clothes smelling fresh and clean.

Safe Use of Essential Oils

Essential oils are the concentrated essences of plants. They seem relatively harmless at first glance, but that small vial you're holding in your hand may have taken hundreds, if not thousands, of plants to produce. It's easy to underestimate their true power because they're easy to obtain and it seems like everyone is talking about them these days. I've seen people hand their teenage kids a vial of essential oil, who then proceeded to pour it onto their arms and rub it in to relieve pain from sore muscles. When I asked what they were using, the girls told me it was a blend of frankincense and a couple other oils. I cringed because this sort of application can cause all kinds of different problems.

When it comes to safe use of essential oils, a small amount of oil goes a long way. For oils that are safe for neat application, a couple drops of oil are all that's needed. Oils that need to be diluted can be added a few drops at a time to a tablespoon of carrier oil to create oil blends that's more than potent enough for most situations. Any more than that and the skin can be burnt, especially if hot oils are used. It may not happen the first time, but wonton use of essential oils can result in sensitization and a skin reaction can occur that precludes the sufferer of the reaction from ever using those essential oils again.

Keep essential oils put away where they're out of the reach of children. Most essential oils are too strong for younger children. If you decide to use essential oils on your older children, it should always be done under your supervision and the oils should always be diluted.

Be aware that essential oils are highly flammable and need to be kept away from open flames.

People who have health problems and/or are taking medications need to consult with their physician prior to beginning use of essential oils. Certain oils can interact with certain types of medication and the reaction could negate or amplify the effects of the medication. Pregnant women should avoid using most essential oils because there are certain oils that can bring on menstruation and uterine contractions. Unless you're sure an oil is safe, it's best to avoid it altogether while pregnant or attempting to get pregnant.

When you add a new oil to your collection, it's important to make sure you research that oil and learn about the potential problems that could arise when you use it. Always start by heavily diluting the oil and testing it in a small area before applying it to larger areas of your body. This is an important step for everyone, but those with sensitive skin need to be particularly cautious. Wait 24 hours after application before applying more oil.

If you're making oil blends, skin care products, bath melts or anything else that requires working with essential oils for a long period of time, make sure you're working in a well-ventilated area. Prolonged exposure to certain oils can have a narcotic effect, and this effect can be amplified if you're in a poorly-ventilated room with little air circulation.

Ingested essential oils can be toxic to the body. If oil is accidentally ingested, contact your local Poison Control Center for directions on the best course of action. I know there are some resources out there that recommend ingesting certain oils, but this is rarely a good idea. The other methods of application are safer and the oils make it into the body without having to pass through the digestive system, where they can be damaged by stomach acids and rendered ineffective.

Diluting Essential Oil with Carrier Oils

Most essential oils are too powerful to be applied directly to the skin at full strength. They can burn the skin and may cause sensitization, which is a reaction that results in the inability to use that particular oil again without irritation. Sensitization can make it so you can't use the oil again even if it's diluted. Redness, itching, burning and even blistering can come about as a result of the skin reacting negatively to essential oil.

Negative reactions are more common with oils known as *hot oils*, which are oils that contain compounds that heat up the skin and the tissue beneath it. Hot oils can cause skin irritation even when they're diluted, but the chance of irritation increases greatly when they're applied at full strength. It's considered a best practice to always test a new essential oil by adding a tiny amount of oil to carrier oil and rubbing it into an inconspicuous area of the skin. Wait 24 hours to see if there's a reaction, and if there is, discontinue use of the oil immediately.

Mild nut and vegetable oils that are primarily made of fats can be used as *carrier oils* to dilute the more potent essential oils and carry them beneath the surface of the skin. Since there are very few people who have a negative reaction to carrier oil, a few drops of essential oil can be blended into a tablespoon of carrier oil and applied topically. Different people prefer different carrier oils, so experiment to see which carrier oils you prefer.

The following oils are all thought to be good carrier oils:

- **Apricot kernel oil.** Inexpensive oil that has a nutty fragrance that smells like apricots. It works great for dry skin.
- **Avocado oil.** Smells nutty and sweet. It works great on dry, cracked skin because it leaves behind a protective coating. Blend a small amount of this oil into other oils for best results.
- **Coconut oil.** This is one of the top carrier oils. It's inexpensive, works well with most skin types and can be used to disperse essential oils into water.
- **Grapeseed oil.** Made from the seeds of grapes, this oil smells light and nutty. It's an inexpensive oil that works well for most skin types.
- **Jojoba oil.** Another popular oil, this one's made from the seeds of the jojoba plant. It's really waxy, so it's best when used in small amounts as part of a carrier oil blend. Jojoba oil is a good choice for oily skin.
- **Rosehip seed oil.** This oil is made from rosehips and it's one of the more expensive carrier oils on the market today. It's a good choice for sensitive skin and should be used as a small part of a carrier oil blend.
- **Sunflower seed oil.** This oil leaves the skin feeling soft and supple. It's on the cheaper side and is a good choice for most skin types.
- **Sweet almond oil.** Another good carrier oil for most skin types, sweet almond oil is an inexpensive oil that softens the skin. It leaves

behind a light oily sheen, but is a great budget oil. Don't use sweet almond oil if you're allergic to almonds.

When creating oil blends in cooler weather, some of the oils you're trying to combine might become solids. If this happens, gently heat the oils until they melt and then stir them together. Don't add the essential oils until the carrier oil blend has cooled down.

Stocking Up: 10 Oils You're Going to Need

Starting an essential oil collection can be a daunting task. Go to the typical store that carries essential oils and you'll find as many as 20 to 30 oils from different plants sitting on the shelf. Search online and you'll find sites that have a hundred or more individual oils. Factor in oil blends and you've quite literally got hundreds of different varieties to choose from.

You can diversify your collection with exotic oils later on if you'd like, but when starting out, there are a handful of essential oils you're going to want to have on hand. Stock your medicine cabinet with the 10 essential oils discussed in this chapter and you'll have most of your bases covered from the get-go.

#10: Citronella Essential Oil

Citronella essential oil is steam-distilled from the *Cymbopogon nardus* or *Cymbopogon witerianus* plant, which is a tall perennial grass that's easy to grow and contains essential oil packed full of compounds known as citronellal and geraniol. *Cymbopogon winteranius* is known as Java citronella and contains higher levels of citronellol and geraniol. Because of the elevated levels of those two compounds, it has a stronger smell and is the preferred choice for perfumery. Citronella oil is steam-distilled and has a sweet citrus smell to it with grassy high notes. The citronella plant is native to Sri Lanka, but is also grown in India, Africa, Vietnam and Central and South America.

In addition to being used for aromatherapy purposes, citronella is also found in a number of products, including perfumes, soaps, household cleaners and insect repellent sprays and candles.

The oil of the citronella plant has a number of benefits associated with it, which we'll get to in a bit, but it's rounding out the top 10 essential oils to own for one reason and one reason only. Insects hate the scent of citronella and a whiff of the oil will send them running, flying or crawling in the opposite direction. Add citronella oil to a spray bottle full of water and spray it around the house to repel ants, fleas, moths, roaches and all sorts of insects. It can be diffused into rooms you want to clear of bugs and can even be used outside, but you're going to have to surround the area you want to keep clear of bugs with diffusers or citronella candles. It can also be diluted with carrier oil and applied topically to keep biting insects like mosquitoes and ticks from pestering you while you're out and about.

Combine it with cedarwood oil to double the bug repellent power and really keep the bugs away.

The benefits of citronella oil don't stop at clearing your house of bugs, as it has a number of other properties associated with it. It's antiseptic, antibacterial, diuretic, tonic and has deodorant qualities. It's an emmenagogue oil, so avoid using it while pregnant. Citronella essential oil is also cicatrisant, meaning it can be massaged into scars and stretch marks to help them fade away.

Aromatherapy uses of citronella oil include diffusing it to relieve stress and diluting it and massaging it into painful joints and sore muscles. Citronella oil is a warming oil that produces a gentle heat when properly diluted and applied topically. The fragrance of citronella is considered uplifting and stimulating, and it can be used to fight off nervous stress and to help with headaches and migraines. When added to skin care products, citronella is used to combat excessively oily skin and may be effective in helping eliminate acne.

Citronella oil is considered non-toxic and is safe for most people to use, aside from pregnant women, but there is a small risk of dermal irritation when the oil is applied to the skin. Always dilute it before application and discontinue use if any signs of skin irritation or rash arise.

#9: Frankincense

Most people are at least passively familiar with frankincense oil. It's one of the oldest essential oils known to mankind and, along with myrrh, was one of the essential oils the wise men brought as gifts for baby Jesus when they traveled to see him upon his birth. It was also found in none other than King Tut's tomb, which should come as no surprise since frankincense was once one of the most sought-after and treasured essential oils in the world.

There are several species of trees from which frankincense can be acquired, the most common of which are *Boswellia carterii* and *Boswellia sacra*. Frankincense acquired from *Boswellia sacra* trees is commonly referred to as sacred frankincense, while the oil from *Boswellia carterii* trees is simply called frankincense. While there are slight differences in the fragrance and chemical composition of oils drawn from these two trees, they're close enough to where they have similar benefits. They both contain large amounts of limonene and pinene, along with a number of other beneficial constituents. In addition to the aforementioned species, frankincense oil is obtained from a number of other *Boswellia* trees, and can vary in quality from great to far below aromatherapy standards. Because of the cost and the time it takes to obtain the resin, this is one of the oils that's often adulterated.

Frankincense essential oil is typically steam-distilled from the resin of the trees, the collection of which isn't an easy process, so the oil is priced in the mid- to high-end of the essential oil price spectrum. It's often used as a base note in perfume blends thanks to its deep, spicy balsamic fragrance that carries the slightest hint of citrus on the top end.

There are a number of therapeutic properties associated with frankincense essential oil. It's analgesic and lends itself well to being diluted with carrier oil and massaged into tender muscles and aching joints. Frankincense oil is beneficial to dry, aging skin thanks to its regenerative properties and can be used to fade scars, wrinkles and stretch marks. It's also strongly antibacterial and antifungal, and has antioxidant, astringent, carminative, diuretic and sedative properties, and is said to give the immune system a helping hand.

When diffused or added to a sink full of hot water and inhaled, frankincense can be used to break up congestion and to ease respiratory conditions. I've even heard of it being put to use by people who have trouble breathing due to asthma and by those who have bronchitis, but be sure to consult with your physician prior to use. If steam inhalation doesn't work, try applying the oil to a hot compress and placing it on your chest.

On a spiritual level, frankincense helps center the emotions and focus the mind, making it a great oil for meditation. It can be used to awaken one's spiritual awareness and may play a key role in improving the ability to overcome distress, sadness and despair. The fragrance of frankincense oil is soothing and relaxing, but not so much so that it makes you drowsy like some of the stronger sedative oils. A light misting of frankincense oil blended with water into a room will leave the room free of odor and it will still smell great hours later.

While it's safe for most people to use, frankincense oil should be diluted before topical application. Consult with your physician prior to using this oil if you're pregnant or have a medical condition.

#8: Eucalyptus Oil

Growing up, I was lucky enough to live near a eucalyptus grove, and my mother would make a point of going there on occasion just to walk through the grove and breathe deeply of the woody, campherous smell of eucalyptus. She didn't know anything about essential oils or aromatherapy, but she knew she liked the way she felt when she walked through the grove, breathing deeply and taking in the scent.

Eucalyptus essential oil is extracted from a variety of different varieties of eucalyptus trees, the most-used of which is *Eucalyptus globulus*. The oil is usually steam-distilled from the leaves and twigs of the tree and is clear and of a consistency similar to that of water. For the uninitiated, eucalyptus is a special treat. It has a fresh, medicinal fragrance thanks to the cineol, camphene and pinene in the oil. Most people who smell eucalyptus for the first time compare it to vapor rub.

The therapeutic properties of eucalyptus oil are many and include the oil being analgesic, antibacterial, anti-inflammatory, antiseptic, antispasmodic, antiviral, astringent, cicatrisant, decongestant, expectorant, rubifacient, purifying and stimulant.

Eucalyptus oil has a cooling effect and opens up the airways, which makes it a good choice for allergy relief, mild fevers, flus and the common cold. It can be rubbed into the chest to help clear up congestion and coughing and diffused eucalyptus oil is great for clearing up congestion of the sinuses and lungs.

While eucalyptus oil produces a cooling sensation upon application, it's actually a warming oil with rubifacient properties that can be used to improve poor circulation and may provide relief from aches and pains in both joints and muscles. It can be diluted and used as a skin care oil that's effective on acne, burns, blisters, minor cuts and scrapes, insect bites and skin infections.

Eucalyptus essential oil has a number of external applications and is a great oil to have on-hand because of its broad range of abilities, but only when small amounts of the oil are applied topically or diffused. Extra care should be taken to ensure eucalyptus oil is properly diluted and it should never be ingested because it can be toxic when large amounts are used. Because of their lighter weight, smaller children are especially susceptible to eucalyptus oil, so make sure it's always put away somewhere that it's out of the reach of younger hands.

#7: Lemon Oil

While there were a handful of citrus oils like grapefruit oil and bergamot oil that could have made the top 10, I settled on lemon oil because of its fresh scent and its ability to be blended with almost any other oil out there to good effect. Lemon oil comes from the peel of lemons. If you want to see what it smells like, all you have to do is bend a lemon peel back and forth a few times. The little jets of liquid that erupt from the peel are lemon essential oil. The oil contains large amounts of limonene and citral, which gives it the characteristic lemon-fresh scent we've all come to associate with lemons.

There are a ton of therapeutic properties attributed to lemon oil. It's antimicrobial, antibacterial and antifungal, which means it works well when diluted and applied to fungal or bacterial infections. It can also be used combat colds and the flu. Lemon oil is rubifacient, so it can be used to improve circulation and may even help temporarily lower blood pressure. Add a drop or two of lemon oil to a bandage before covering cuts, scrapes, burns and blisters and they'll heal faster and with less scarring.

When diffused, lemon essential oil is a great room deodorizer that leaves the room it's diffused in smelling clean and fresh. Diffused lemon oil has stimulant properties and can be used to lift your spirits when you're feeling burnt out or down in the dumps.

Natural home cleaning products are frequently scented with lemon essential oil. It doesn't just leave the surfaces it comes in contact with smelling nice and clean; it's a potent one-two punch that eliminates harmful microorganisms and helps keep them away.

Lemon oil is a powerful oil and it can be a dermal irritant to those with sensitive skin. It's also phototoxic, which means it can cause skin irritation when an area of the skin lemon oil was applied to is exposed to the sun within 24 hours of application.

#6: Geranium Oil

Geranium oil is steam-distilled from the flowers and leaves of the geranium plant. The oil ranges in color from dark yellow to greenish yellow, and while it might be a bit disconcerting to get different colors from different suppliers, there's little discernible difference between the colors. They all have a similar floral fragrance, with some being slightly mintier than others. The main chemical constituents of geranium oil are citronellol, which you probably remember from the chapter on citronella, and geraniol.

Rose geranium oil is a more expensive variety that smells of roses. If you prefer the smell of rose geranium, you can spend the extra cash, but most people get along just fine with regular geranium essential oil unless they need the rose oil to perfect a perfume blend. Dab a drop or two of either of the oils onto your wrists before heading out for the day and you'll smell like you're wearing expensive perfume.

Most people appreciate the smell of geranium oil and look for reasons to use it. Luckily, there's ample opportunity to use this oil thanks to its many benefits. It has analgesic, antibacterial, anti-inflammatory, astringent, cicatrisant, deodorant, rubifacient, sedative and tonic qualities. Geranium oil is diuretic, meaning it increases the rate at which the body produces urine. This can help detoxify the body, but you've got to make sure you drink enough water to help it along. It can be diffused to combat asthma and other respiratory conditions and can be used to clear up congestion and a stuffy head. The fragrance of geranium oil improves emotional stability while enhancing feelings of joy and bringing on a better mood. If you're already happy, it will probably make you happier and may even be able to lift you out of a melancholy mood.

Geranium oil has regenerative properties, which makes it one of the better oils for helping to heal wounds, cuts, scrapes, burns and insect bites, and it can be used to help fade away scars from previous injuries. It's well-suited to all skin types and can be diluted and massaged into the skin to take care of skin problems like acne, eczema, rashes, dermatitis and shingles.

Some people may suffer from skin irritation when geranium oil is applied topically. Pregnant women and children should avoid use of this oil. While it's safe for most other people to dilute and apply it topically or to inhale the fragrance of the oil, it should not be taken internally. A large enough internal dose of this oil can be toxic.

#5: Peppermint

Most people are familiar with the scent of peppermint. The essential oil comes from the peppermint plant, which is a cross between spearmint and water mint, and smells pretty much the same as peppermint candy or chewing gum, but is stronger and has a crisper aroma. Peppermint oil is used to flavor foods, chewing gum and some beverages, so you've probably tasted real peppermint oil before as part of a recipe. Be aware that while peppermint oil is a great oil to have around because of its many uses, it's the most powerful oil on this list and is one you're going to want to be very careful with. A little bit of peppermint oil goes a long way and you don't want to apply too much peppermint oil to your skin...or forget to wash your hands and accidentally touch a sensitive area of your body. Trust me on this one. It probably won't do any lasting damage, but it's an experience you won't soon forget.

Peppermint essential oil gets its characteristic fragrance and much of its power from a chemical compound known as menthol. If you've ever used Vick's Vapor Rub, you've experienced the power of menthol. Peppermint oil has a similar effect, albeit it's more powerful in its undiluted form.

The benefits associated with peppermint oil are many and include it being analgesic, antibacterial, anti-inflammatory, antifungal, antimicrobial, antiseptic, astringent, carminative, cholagogue, expectorant and nervine.

Diffuse peppermint essential oil in small amounts to improve clarity of mind, focus and to help with concentration. In smaller doses, it's stimulant by nature, but can have a sedative effect if you use too much. In addition to providing mental stimulation, diffused peppermint oil is one of the go-to oils for breaking up congestion and providing relief from respiratory conditions. It can be diffused or steam containing the oil can be inhaled, or it can be diluted and applied directly to the chest. Another use for diffused peppermint oil is for eliminating headaches and making migraines more tolerable. It probably won't completely eliminate a migraine, but it might bring it down a decibel or two, which is all I can hope for some days.

Dilute it with carrier oil and apply it topically and peppermint oil produces a cooling sensation in the area where it's applied. What you're actually feeling is the oil stimulating the nerves. It feels cool at first and gradually starts to warm up as the capillaries open and blood starts to flow. This effect can be used to relieve muscle spasms, muscles pains, joint pains and pain associated with arthritis.

Children, those who are epileptic and pregnant women should not use peppermint oil. It's considered a hot oil and there's the potential for a serious skin reaction or sensitization, especially if the oil isn't used properly. Dilute it before applying it topically for best results. If you still can't handle peppermint oil even after it's been diluted, spearmint essential oil is milder and may be a better choice.

Mix a few drops into a cup of water and use it as mouthwash to eliminate bad breath and fight the germs that cause cavities, but stop short of actually swallowing it. There are a number of sources that indicate peppermint oil is safe for consumption in small amounts. It can be neurotoxic if you consume too much, so only go this route under the supervision of a medical professional.

Insects and small rodents don't care for the smell of peppermint oil, so it can be used as a natural deterrent. Make a bug repellent spray by mixing 10 drops of peppermint oil into a spray bottle full of water and spray it everywhere you don't want bugs. It works on bug bites as well. Rub a drop into a bug bite to immediately kill the itching or dab it onto a bee sting to eliminate the pain.

#4: Oregano Oil

Oregano essential oil is steam-distilled from the flowering plant of the oregano herb, which is the same herb that's used to add flavor to culinary dishes across the globe. I love that the oil smells similar to the spice and has the same warm, herbaceous fragrance. There are a wide variety of oregano essential oils on the market today. Look for oil that's high in carvacrol for best results.

Properties associated with oregano oil include it being analgesic, antibacterial, antifungal, antimicrobial, antiseptic, antispasmodic, antiviral, carminative, cholagogue, emmenagogue and expectorant.

When I first feel an illness starting to come on, I diffuse oregano oil into the air to take advantage of its antiviral properties. I can't say for sure that it works, but it seems like I'm sick less often than I used to be and the times I am sick are of shorter duration. Oregano oil can help when you're stuffed up or congested if you inhale the fragrance or rub diluted oil onto your chest. It's naturally anti-inflammatory and may help soothe inflamed tissue in the lungs and ease coughing fits. The anti-inflammatory properties can also be used to help ease symptoms associated with seasonal allergies.

Dilute oregano oil with carrier oil and apply it topically to get rid of athlete's foot, nail fungus and other fungal infections, along with a variety of rashes and skin conditions. It can also be used to speed up muscle recovery and to dull aches and pains.

Oil of oregano is emmenagogue, so it should be avoided by pregnant women. While this is not a good oil to use while expecting, it can be used to ease the effects of painful periods and irregular menstruation. Since it's a very potent warming oil, it can irritate sensitive skin and needs to be diluted before topical application. Always test it in a small area first prior to applying it to a larger area.

Yet another use for oregano oil is to dilute it with water and spray it onto areas you want to clean and disinfect. It removes a number of harmful microorganisms and may even fight salmonella and E. coli.

#3: German Chamomile

We're headed into the top 3 essential oils you should own when embarking on your journey. If you don't have the money to buy all the oils on the list at once, these three oils can be purchased and will cover a variety of situations. This spot was a toss-up between Roman chamomile, which comes from *Chamaemeleum nobile*, and German chamomile, which is obtained from the *Matricaria recutita* plant. Both oils are great oils to own, but I settled upon German chamomile over Roman chamomile because it contains large amounts of chamazulene, which ups the health factor and gives it a pretty blue color.

German chamomile is analgesic, antiallergenic, antibacterial, antibiotic, anti-inflammatory, antispasmodic, carminative, emmenagogue, sedative, vermifuge and vulnerary. It can be diffused into a room for stress relief and the soothing fragrance of the oil may provide headache and migraine relief. It's a calming oil that can be used when it's time to relax and wind down.

One of the biggest benefits of German chamomile is its ability to eliminate skin conditions like eczema, pruritus and skin infections. It knocks down both internal and external inflammation and speeds up the healing process when applied to wounds, cuts, scrapes, burns and insect bites. It's also effective against gout and can provide relief from arthritis pain, sore muscles and joint pain.

German chamomile is safe for most people to use, but the chamazulene in the oil might irritate sensitive skin. Those who are allergic to ragweed should steer clear of German chamomile because it can provoke a similar immune response. Always test it on a small area prior to applying it to a larger swath of skin.

#2: Tea Tree Oil

Tea tree oil is like the Swiss Army knife of essential oils. If I was forced to choose only one essential oil to use for the rest of my life, it would probably be tea tree oil. It's really that powerful. Tea tree oil is steam distilled from the leaves and twigs of the tea tree, known to the scientific community as *Melaleuca alternifolia*. The oil has a medicinal, herbaceous scent to it that most people don't care for the first time they inhale it. Don't worry...Once you've used it a few times, you'll learn to love it.

The oil of the tea tree is analgesic, antibacterial, antifungal, anti-inflammatory, antimicrobial, antiparasitic, antiviral, decongestant, deodorant, diaphoretic, stimulant and vulnerary. It's also got insect repellent properties and can be used in lieu of citronella, but isn't quite as powerful.

When diluted and applied topically, tea tree oil is a soothing oil that reduces inflammation and promotes the healing of damaged skin. Combine it with aloe vera and rub it into a sunburn to ease the pain and to help prevent blistering. It heals skin infections and some people use it to help reduce and eliminate acne. If you've got an itching or burning rash or chickenpox, tea tree oil can provide relief. It antifungal and can be used on athlete's foot, nail fungus and on other fungal infections.

Tea tree oil lends itself well to dental health care products. Add a few drops to a cup full of water and use it as mouthwash to eliminate the bacteria that cause cavities and bad breath and to keep your mouth smelling clean. It can also be added to natural toothpaste recipes to provide an added boost.

Create an all-purpose cleaner that cleans and disinfects naturally by adding 15 to 20 drops of tea tree oil to a spray bottle full of water. This cleaner can be used to clean most hard surfaces and is a great choice for cleaning toilets, sinks, cutting boards and spraying into smelly refrigerators. This same spray can be sprayed on areas where ants or other insects are entering the house to keep them outside where they belong. Add a few drops of tea tree oil to your pets collar to drive away fleas and ticks.

Applying tea tree oil topically is safe for most people, but it can cause skin irritation and possibly sensitization. The chance of a reaction increases when the oil is applied neat, which many people opt to do. Do not take tea tree oil orally and make sure you spit it out when using it as part of your dental care routine.

#1: Lavender

I'm not breaking any new ground by choosing lavender oil as the number one essential oil you're going to want to own. Most lists of popular essential oils have lavender pegged at number one. It's one of the most versatile oils around, it's inexpensive to buy, and it's one of the more mild and forgiving oils. Most people are able to apply it to their skin neat without experiencing any irritation whatsoever and it carries with it a number of therapeutic and mental benefits.

It's important to make sure you're buying the right kind of lavender oil or you might end up losing a lot of its potency right out the box. True lavender oil is distilled from the *Lavandula augustifolia* plant. Don't get lavender oil mixed up with spike lavender oil, which is a different plant altogether. Lavandin oil is another oil that's commonly confused with lavender oil. It contains lavender oil, but is actually a blend of lavender oil and spike lavender oil.

Lavender essential oil carries with it a number of therapeutic qualities, including being analgesic, anticonvulsant, antidepressant, antihistamine, anti-inflammatory, antimicrobial, antiseptic, antitumor, antiviral, calming, deodorant, relaxing and soothing. It works well for healing cuts, scrapes, burns, bruises, skin rashes, sunburns and all sorts of other minor skin conditions. In fact, the healing capabilities of lavender oil were discovered when a French scientist name René Gattefossé burnt his hand and dipped it into lavender oil for relief. It didn't just ease the pain. His hand healed quickly and with minimal scarring.

The fragrance of lavender oil has calming and soothing properties and it will calm the mind and ease any troubled emotions you may be having. Diffuse the oil into a room or rub a few drops between your palms and hold it up to your nose and mouth to inhale the fragrance. The calming effect will bring you back down to earth when you're wound up and can be used to help you relax enough to where you're ready to fall asleep at night.

Lavender oil has insect repellent properties and can be used to repel moths, fleas, flies, bees and ants. It isn't as powerful as some of the other insect repellent oils like citronella and peppermint oil, but it's a heck of a lot milder and is safer to apply to older children and teenagers.

Essential Oil Blends

Essential oils are powerful when taken at face value, but combining them will place even more powerful concoctions at your fingertips. It only takes a minute or two to create an oil blend and you're able to combine the effects of a number of oils into a single potent blend. It's important to carefully consider the oils you're adding to an oil blend because it's all too easy to combine oils and end up with a blend that has properties you didn't want to add.

Here are the steps I recommend when deciding which oils you'd like to blend together:

1. **Look for essential oils that have the properties you desire.** For example, if you have a cold, you're going to want to look for oils that have decongestant and expectorant properties. If your body aches all over, you're also going to need oils that work for aches and pains. Antiviral and antibacterial oils can help ease the duration of the cold, especially if used early on, so add those to the list as well. Got a headache? Add oils that eliminate headaches to the list, too. Once you've got a list of oils you're considering and their properties, move onto step 2.
2. **Look for the oils that cover a number of the problems you're trying to solve.** If you're only trying to solve one problem, look for oils that work best to eliminate or ease that problem. These should be your top contenders.

3. **Look at the other properties of the oils and eliminate oils that have undesirable effects.** For example, if you're looking for oils that help ease the effects of the cold, but it's getting late at night and you're ready for bed, you'll want to eliminate oils that have a stimulant effect because they might keep you awake. If you're pregnant or trying to get pregnant, oils that have emmenagogue properties should be crossed off the list. Other considerations that need to be made is possible interactions with medications you're taking and the effect the oil is going to have based on your current medical condition.

4. **Consider how the remaining oils are going to smell when combined.** This is one of the tougher things for beginners to take in because there's a lot to consider. More on this in a bit.

5. **Combine the essential oils.** If you're creating a new oil blend, you can combine a few drops of each of the oils to test them out. Make sure you keep track of what you've added to the oil blend or you run the risk of creating a blend you love, but aren't able to replicate. If you're creating a blend you're already familiar with, you can combine more oil, so you'll have it available when you want it.

6. **Place them into an airtight glass container and let them sit overnight.** This is the hardest part. Don't judge your oil blend right away because the oils need time to meld together and

mature. Wait a day or two before smelling your blend and deciding whether you like it or not.

Not too bad, right? Blending essential oils is easy when all you're concerned with are the therapeutic benefits of the oils. It gets much more complicated when you start worrying about the fragrance of the oil blend in addition to the benefits.

Categories and Notes: Creating Fragrant Oil Blends

While you could simply blend essential oils based on their therapeutic properties alone and end up with oil blends that smell halfway decent and work well, it's preferable that you have at least a passing knowledge of how the fragrances are going to combine with one another. This will allow you to look at the essential oils you're considering using and decide which of the oils will probably combine the best. Keep in mind that much of what you're going to learn in this chapter boils down to personal preference, so it's going to take some experimentation on your part to decide what sort of oil blends you like the best.

It's part science, part art and a whole lot of experimentation. Take the time to learn the ins and outs of blending fragrances and you'll be able to come up with oil blends that are amazing.

There are three key considerations that must be made when creating essential oil blends:

- **The effect of the oil.**
- **The category the oil falls into.**
- **The note of the oil.**

We already discussed looking at the effect of the oil in the previous chapter. Once you've determined which essential oils best suit your needs, it's time to start looking at how the different oils will combine and that's determined by the category and the note.

The *category* of the oil is the grouping into which an essential oil is placed based on a decision made by looking at both the type of plant the oil came from and the fragrance the oil has. Here are the categories essential oils are divided into:

- **Campherous oils.** Campherous oils like eucalyptus and tea tree oil have the medicinal fragrance of camphor. They're strong oils that can easily overpower lighter oils in a blend if you aren't careful.
- **Citrus oils.** These oils have the light smell of citrus. They include orange, bergamot, lime, grapefruit and lemon essential oil.
- **Floral oils.** Floral oils are derived from flowers and smell like the flowers they were distilled from. Popular floral oils include geranium, rose and lavender oil.
- **Herb oils.** These oils are taken from and smell like the herbs that are used for cooking and include popular herbs like basil, oregano and rosemary.
- **Mint oils.** These oils have the unmistakable fragrance of mint. Spearmint and peppermint are two of the more common mint oils.
- **Spice oils.** These oils are referred to as Oriental or exotic oils in some literature. They have unmistakable fragrances that are unlike any other essential oil. Oils like patchouli and ylang ylang oil are classified as spice oils.

- **Wood oils.** These oils are taken from trees. They smell fresh and woodsy and sometimes feature a campherous fragrance. Pine, cedarwood and eucalyptus oil are all tree oils.

Blending oils based on the category they're in is more art than it is science, so you can place oils in the different categories based on the fragrance you detect when you smell them. As you can see, there is some overlap between the groupings. For example, eucalyptus oil could be classified as either wood oil, because it's taken from trees, or campherous oil because of its fragrance. I would personally place it into the campherous category, but a pretty good argument could be made that it's a wood oil.

Here are some basic rules to follow when blending essential oils:

- **Wood oils can be blended with most other oils to good effect.**
- **Campherous oils are tough to blend with other oils because they tend to overpower oil blends.** If you do decide to blend them, use small amounts of the campherous oil and larger amounts of the other oils.
- **Floral oils combine well with spice oils and citrus oils.** They also work well with some wood oils.
- **Citrus oils can be used to add the light fragrance of citrus to most oil blends, but they tend to work best with floral oils or herb oils.**

- **Mint oils blend well with citrus oils, but can quickly overpower a blend.**

Of course, you know what they say about rules—they were made to be broken. Some of my favorite oils blends ignore the previous rules altogether and came about as a result of me thinking, "I wonder what would happen if I blended [oil A] with [oil B]." It doesn't always work, but as long as you only blend small amounts of oil, your experimental blends won't be too expensive and you can either use them quickly or throw them out.

The next consideration that must be made is the *note* of the oil, which is a classification of the oil based on how long the fragrance of the oil lasts. There are three basic notes:

- **Base notes.** These are the heaviest fragrances and they stick around the longest. Base notes are notes you'll still smell hours after application. Spice oils and some wood oils are classified as base notes.
- **Middle notes.** Heavy notes, but not quite as heavy as base notes. They're the bridge between the top notes and the base notes. All of the categories contain at least a few oils that are classified as middle notes.
- **Top notes.** These are the first notes you smell in an oil blend. Top notes are light, and they dance around your nose and quickly dissipate. Top notes are scattered throughout the categories. Most of the citrus oils are considered top notes.

The way notes work is the first fragrance you smell in a blend is the top note combined with the other notes. It's a light note that quickly dissipates, leaving you with the middle and base notes. The middle note is often the defining note of a blend because it provides the bridge between the top note and the base note. Once the middle note has dissipated, you're left with the base note, which can last a long time after you apply an oil blend.

Don't forget to factor in the smell of any carrier oils you plan on using. Most carrier oils won't add a lot of fragrance, but they may add a slight nutty or fruity aroma to the mix.

Essential Oil Blends to Try

Blending essential oils is fun, but when first starting out it can be a bit daunting. The oil blends in this section are all designed to get you off to a good start, but aren't the end-all, be-all of essential oil blending. Use them as they are or feel free to modify them to suit your tastes. These blends use only the 10 oils from the "Stocking Up" chapter to create a number of effects. When you think about it, it's amazing how versatile essential oils really are.

These recipes are all best-suited for diffusion or being diluted and applied topically. They might work in candles, bath bombs, skin care products and for other applications, but they haven't been tested.

I used *parts* as the unit of measurement for the recipes. In order to use the recipes, all you have to do is substitute

The Cold Buster

1 part peppermint oil + 2 parts lavender oil + 1 part eucalyptus oil

If you're congested or feeling stuffed up, a few whiffs of this oil blend might be all it takes to ease the symptoms of your cold or seasonal allergies. This oil blend works best when you add it to a sink full of hot water and inhale the steam. It can also be diluted with carrier oil and rubbed onto your chest, but it might get a little warm!

The Floral Happiness Blend

1 part geranium oil + 1 part lavender oil + 1 part German chamomile

This blend will leave rooms it's diffused into smelling like a flower garden. What more could you want?

The Good Morning Blend

2 parts lemon oil + 1 part peppermint oil

If you've got a long day ahead and want to start it off right, this is a great oil blend to diffuse into the kitchen while you have breakfast. You'll feel wide awake and alert after a few minutes.

Fresh Air

1 part lavender oil + 1 part lemon oil + 1 part oregano oil

This blend takes 3 essential oils that can be used on their own to freshen the air in a room and combines them to create a great-smelling blend that will eliminate even the toughest of odors. Diffuse it into a room or add it to a spray bottle full of water and mist it on items you want to destink.

Detox

1 part geranium oil + 1 part peppermint oil + 1 part citronella oil

The Detox blend works on multiple levels. It aids the digestive systems and helps the body eliminate toxins. It can be added to a bath you're soaking in or it can be diluted and applied topically.

The Bug Blaster

1 part peppermint oil + 1 part citronella oil + 1 part eucalyptus oil

This blend is hell on wheels when it comes to eliminating bugs, but I've got to warn you. It's extremely potent and must be diluted heavily prior to topical application. Even then, you might not be able to tolerate it.

The Back to Earth Blend

1 part frankincense oil + 1 part German chamomile oil

When you're wound up and your emotions are on the verge of getting the best of you, the Back to Earth blend is a grounding blend that will help you corral your emotions. Turn down the lights, sit down and breathe deeply while you diffuse it into the room.

Fever Buster

1 part lemon oil + 1 part lavender oil + 1 part peppermint oil

Dilute this oil and apply it to the forehead, back and neck for fever relief. It should only be used with minor fevers. Bad fevers or fevers that don't let up within a day or two require medical attention.

Anti-Aging Blend

2 parts frankincense oil + 1 part geranium oil

The regenerative properties of both of these oils can be combined to tighten up aging skin and to help reduce wrinkles and skin damage.

The Cleansing Blend

2 parts lemon oil + 1 part citronella oil

Combine these two oils and add them to a spray bottle full of water to create an oil blend that can be used to clean all sorts of hard surfaces. This blend can also be diffused to cleanse the mind and the body.

Aches & Pains

2 parts peppermint essential oil and 1 part German chamomile

Dilute this oil blend with carrier oil and massage it into aching muscles or joints. The analgesic properties will help deaden the area and will provide temporary relief from the pain.

Burns & Wounds

2 parts lavender oil and 1 part tea tree oil

Add this blend to lukewarm water and use it to wash out minor wounds. It can be applied to the bandage prior to covering a wound to promote healing and help prevent scarring.

The End

Thanks again for purchasing (or downloading) this book. I really hope you got the information you were looking for and this is the start of a wonderful journey into the world of essential oils for you.